10 Helpful Hints for Carers

Practical solutions for carers living
with people with dementia

Professor June Andrews
Professor Allan House

This book has been made possible by a bequest from Miss Gilda Massari and her family.
It is published in her memory.

It is based on the literature review, *A Systematic Review of Non-Drug Treatments for Dementia*, by Dr Claire Hulme, Judy Wright, Tom Crocker, Yeme Oluboyede and Allan House.

Contents

Foreword

This little book offers some practical solutions to problems that might occur when you are living with a person with dementia. For much of the time, things will be as they always were. You are living with the same person. You know the sort of thing that makes them feel good and helps them to relax. So you are still the expert. But even an expert needs new ideas sometimes.

The ideas contained in here are those where some research has been done to show that they can make a difference, in cases of stress and distress. So you might find them useful in your own situation.

Most importantly the book contains some information about organisations or services that you can turn to for help, because nothing beats talking to someone else who has experience. The book has been put together by researchers from the University of Leeds and the University of Stirling, and was made possible by a generous donation from the Massari family, who lived through this problem themselves.

About this book

This book has been written for people who live with someone who has dementia. People with dementia themselves will find it interesting and you might want to read it together. *Living with* someone who has dementia may eventually develop into *looking after* the person with dementia.

'I was completely at sea. No one told me what to expect. I just did my best.'

However, many people with dementia say they get annoyed if they are treated differently by those they live with, particularly in the early stages of their condition, so remember that your husband, wife or other loved one is still the person they were yesterday, even though some of the knowledge and experience of their life time may fade away, especially knowledge of more recent things.

The money for the research for this book was given by someone who had to learn the hard way how to cope. Researchers from the University of Leeds were asked to look into the evidence about what works. Writers and teachers from the Dementia Services Development Centre at the University of Stirling were asked to put the research into words.

Not all of the problems described in this book will happen to you. Even if you are experiencing any of them, they may not be a permanent feature.

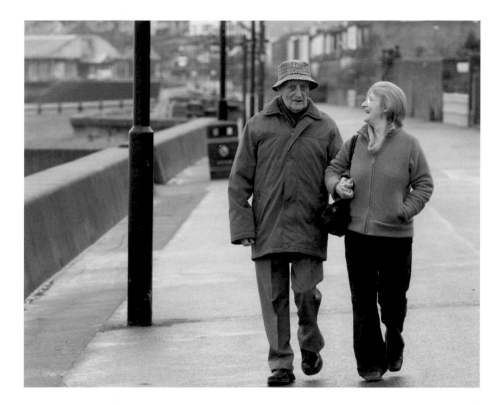

'Henry got very agitated during the second year after he got his diagnosis. He's not like that now, but it was awful while it lasted.'

As well as giving some ideas about how to cope, this book tells you where you might go for further help. We say 'might' because sadly the care for people with dementia is patchy around the country. Some of the things suggested might not work where you live. However, the people you contact in your area will probably be able tell you about good things near you which are not mentioned in this book.

This brings us to the most important advice in the book. You are never alone, no matter how isolated you feel. You are surrounded by a network of health and social care services, and voluntary services which have been specifically set up to help people in your situation. But remember that there are other people in your life who want to help. They can't do that if you hide your problem from them. Family and friends can get involved, and your place of worship or any societies that you are part of, such as Rotary or the WI, will always have among their members people who have already experienced what you are going through.

'I knew Alison had vascular dementia, but it was only when someone said "Ask the Alzheimer's Society" that I realised they deal with any kind of dementia, and they've got a meeting I can go to. I met a man just like me and his wife was the same as Alison. He did make me laugh. He says I made him feel better because he felt less alone. Now his wife has passed away he comes round sometimes and entices me out to the pub. (Not that I need much persuasion!)'

Creating A Relaxing Environment

Every one of the problems listed in the seven sections of this book has ten suggested solutions or helpful hints. Many of them can be solved more easily if the atmosphere is calm and relaxed. If someone is shouting, repeating themselves, refusing to eat, trying to go out in unsuitable clothes (sometimes all at the same time!) staying calm and relaxed would be a miracle. So the secret is to put as much in place as possible to keep a relaxed background environment. This means avoiding over stimulation – and everyone has different things that they find stimulating so you have to decide for yourself what will work in your circumstances. Also remember that stress is infectious. So if any of these things make you as a carer feel good, your relaxed state will help your loved one.

10 helpful hints for a relaxed atmosphere:

1. Get rid of clutter. Imagine the 'before and after' picture. The kitchen surfaces are littered with gadgets and notebooks, postcards and holiday souvenirs. Try to put everything you only use occasionally behind a cupboard door. Only keep out on the surface things that you need every day. For example, your cup and kettle, teabags and biscuit tin should be there on a clear work top. You can label cupboards, or replace the cupboard door with a see-through panel so that the contents can be seen. This means the person with dementia doesn't have to remember where things are and go raking around in drawers and cupboards for them, getting angry and frustrated. Put everything they are unlikely to be looking for in a less prominent place and help them to easily find what they need for themselves.

2. Have more light. Increase the wattage of all the light bulbs in the house and get more fitments if possible. Clean the windows and cut bushes away to let more light in. Push curtains and pelmets right back to get the benefit of daylight. As we age, our eyes get less efficient. If you can't remember where something is, and you are having to look for it, shedding some light on the subject is a very good idea. People with dementia get confused and mistake what they are looking at, if the light is poor. They may think a shadow is a stranger, or that the pattern in the wallpaper is someone looking at them.

3. Sometimes have less light! Think about the lighting conditions which are best for your loved one at night; if they are used to the dark, make the room dark. If they like soft, gentle light at night do that. Be careful to make sure the lighting is flexible. There are movement sensors which are easy to buy that will automatically light up the toilet area when someone gets out of bed. This helps the confused person find the toilet. If you can position their bed so that when they are in the toilet they can see their bed, that helps too, but it isn't possible in every house. Make sure your outside light is off if possible, in case the person goes outside, attracted by the light.

4. Keep the noise down. Shutting doors and windows if there is competing noise can help. Only have the radio or TV on if someone is really listening to it. Having favourite music on can screen unhelpful noise, and it is also relaxing.

Radio music with frequent news or advertising interruptions is less helpful for staying calm.

5. Watch out for mirrors (or reflections from windows after dark). People with dementia don't immediately recognise their own face in a mirror, and the logical conclusion if you see a stranger staring back at you through a glass, is that it is a window, and this nosy intruder is staring in at you as if you shouldn't be there. One carer showed us how he put a little roller blind above the bathroom mirror. He keeps it down, so that if his wife goes in the bathroom 'the window' is covered, and when he wants to shave or look at his handsome face, he can roll it up. When it is dark outside, shut curtains or blinds to avoid a mirror effect.

6. Create a 'den'. Well, we'd all like that, but especially when stressed, a hideaway is nice. One lady described to us how her husband has one room with his favourite books about football and his CDs and a battered old chair. It has a view of the street so he watches the world going past. After lunch she tempts him in there and he often has an afternoon snooze on the sofa, undisturbed by the rest of the household.

7. Make things smell nice. Those in our sixties will remember how as 'hippie' students we used to burn incense sticks. These days you can buy a vast array of incense burners or scented candles. The daughter of a man with dementia has said that she doesn't know if her dad notices the lavender oil but it makes her feel better anyway!

8. Touch is really important. Some families don't touch much. Sons shake hands with fathers, and daughters peck their mothers on the cheek. Now is the time to learn big hugs, and to learn the pleasure of sitting on the sofa beside your mum, stroking her hair, or rubbing some nice cream into her feet and ankles. Give your dad a manicure. If he is enjoying it, don't even think about the fact that ten years ago he'd have thought it was weird. You can go on a course to learn massage techniques, but gentle stroking doesn't need a certificate. (Also, make sure that you try a massage FOR YOURSELF. If you haven't tried it, we suggest you are missing a treat that you will want again and again.)

9. Pat the dog. Amazingly, petting an animal can reduce your blood pressure and caring for it can give all sorts of health benefits. If the person with dementia doesn't speak, they can still communicate, and the dog knows that he is loved, and will come again and again for scratches and pats. Cats are more mysterious, but they all like a comfy place to sit, and they don't mind if what you say to them doesn't make sense. They'll go away if they don't like it. A fish tank is very calming and relaxing, and less demanding than a four legged pet. The person with dementia can express their love and affection to an animal again and again without embarrassment.

10. Exercise. Exercise reduces stress, and a calm atmosphere requires everyone to have lower stress levels. Even if it is quiet, there is soothing music, you can see where everything is, and the cat is looking for a lap to curl up on, everyone in the house will be stressed if there is excess energy to be burned up. The chaos in the home caused by endless attempts to prevent the person with dementia disappearing out the front or back door can often be helped by taking them for a nice long walk. People can walk on their own. One family told us of a satellite tracking device sewn into their mother's handbag. They had to make sure she only had one bag in the house to make sure that was the one she used. Then if there was an indication that she was out and about dangerously late or dangerously far away, they could go and fetch her, tired but happy, from wherever she had gone.

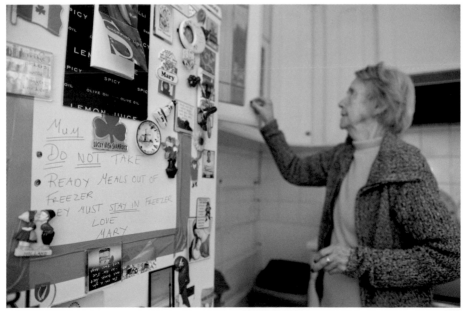

Aggression

People with dementia can become aggressive. It is not your fault, but the result of their condition. Not everyone does, and sometimes it is only over a limited period of time, but it is always horrible, because it hurts the people who are doing most to help. If you have never faced this problem, don't worry about this chapter. It might be upsetting to consider these possibilities, and it might never happen. But it is really important to keep yourself safe, and you must not tolerate it if violence is used against you. You need to get help. If your relationship is with someone who was always aggressive, this is a different and difficult case and you definitely should be asking for help, firstly from your GP. Your psychiatrist can tell you if they have the sort of dementia that is likely to make a person more aggressive. This means you can anticipate problems, and let the health team know if they become an issue.

There are reasons for aggressive behaviour which are to do with the fact that the person has memory and reasoning problems.

• They might be having hallucinations. What would you do if you were alone in the house with your husband, and you heard someone's voice saying 'I think I'll poison her...' just as he walks into the room to offer you a cup of tea. You might throw it back at him.

• They might be very anxious. You are heading for the bathroom with your mum who has soiled her pants, and suddenly she feel unsure about why you are taking off her clothes, and she fights to keep them on. You persist in trying because she can't stay like this, and she scratches your face and pulls your hair in a desperate attempt to fight you off.

• Fear can be an issue. Just imagine how you would feel if you found yourself by the front door facing a stranger in her fifties who insists she is your daughter. But you know your little daughter is at the school gate waiting for you to bring her home! You would be afraid of this mad woman and you might hit her to get away from her and get down to the school. When you have dementia, you may be living in the past and will react aggressively to protect your child.

• Anger and frustration cause violence. You know you were always able to work the TV and now it just won't switch on no matter what buttons you push. So you go to your workshop, find the hammer and just bash the useless object and throw the bits in the bin.

In summary, the aggressive behaviour is an understand-able response from a person who misinterprets what is happening, because of deficits in their understanding and memory. They know something is going wrong and they are angry and scared. So they fight. If you see the world from their point of view, you'd see why it actually makes sense to fight.

10 helpful hints to cope with aggression:

1. Leave the room. Giving the person time and space to calm down is helpful. Especially if you can't work out what went wrong, you remove any possible irritation that you have caused by what you said or did, or how you said or did it. It also means that you are safer. Even if it is limited to verbal aggression, you can't go on being shouted at without it affecting you. It might not have been you that caused it, but try backing off and if this does not help you know you have a more complex situation to deal with. It also removes you from the understandable, but completely unacceptable, temptation to hit them back. It gives you, the carer, time and space to calm down, and even ask for help.

2. Ask yourself if they might be in pain. A lot of the conditions that are common in older age are painful, and the person with dementia might be unable to identify the pain and work out what to do about it. The person might be having any other sort of discomfort, like having a sore tummy with constipation, a pain down below caused by a bladder infection, or a headache, Normally, as adults, we are able to do something to deal with discomfort, but the person with dementia sometimes can't. They might be sitting there, just bearing it, and you come along and cheerfully place their lunch in front of them. If the person throws the tray to the floor, it might be nothing to do with you, or the food.

3. Using touch and calming words can help. Even if what they have said is abusive, unfair or untrue, this is not the time to defend your reputation. Apologise and try to gently stroke an arm or hand. Make sure that when you gently take their hand or put your arm round them it is not in a way that makes them feel as if you are trying to restrain them. The biggest danger with restraining someone is the superhuman effort they will make to get away, perhaps hurting both you and themself in the process.

4. Think of going for a walk. Regular exercise helps to reduce aggression, using up spare energy and acting as a distraction from difficult behaviour. It can provide social activity and routine and structure to the day. It works for both the carer and the person with dementia, and you might even find a friend who is happy to take your loved one (and the dog) for a walk, giving you a break for yourself.

5. Work out what sort of thing gives rise to outbursts. If going for a bath is threatening, check for mirrors or reflections. A shiny bathroom floor can seem wet and slippy, even if it is as dry as a bone. The person will fight back and resist having to walk there. If they are not sure who you are at this moment, they are certainly NOT going to want to take their clothes off, or have you take them off. Giving the person with dementia something to hold may stop them clinging on to their clothes. Nice smells and bubble bath, and gentle music to make it a pleasant experience rather than a wash and scrub up, can aid cooperation. And a major question is... why are you bothering with a bath in the first place? We lived for years in our youth having one bath a week and only if we really needed it. Think about whether it is really necessary now. Sometimes doing less is better.

6. Music was mentioned earlier as background noise to soothe the soul, and to cancel out frightening or extraneous noise that might add to confusion. There are specialist therapists who can provide music therapy and you could ask about those activities from your local Alzheimer's organisation. Playing favourite music has a really positive effect. There is great benefit from enjoying music in groups. Singing together, playing instruments together – any social activity seems to help, and if music is included it has an added positive effect. You can buy CDs of familiar songs to sing along with, including old hymns learned at school and seasonal favourites like Christmas songs. If you can find a musician who will come and share their live music with a group of people with dementia it is great, especially if the musician is good at interacting with the audience and doesn't mind a bit of singing along, heckling and other popular types of involvement. Imagine the pleasure for a person with dementia, who has been getting everything wrong all day, if they are the only person in the room who can sing all five verses of Auld Lang Syne. (You know you'll love it, and you can always wear ear plugs.) If the person with dementia is no longer in the land of their birth, there

may be a club where expatriates can get together and sing familiar songs and share music. This can include Polish and Ukranian clubs, Chinese day centres, or national groups organised around religious faith groups.

7. Make life less boring. You can't turn your home into a holiday camp, and you probably have a significant burden of domestic chores, some of which you used to share, but anything that you can do to relieve boredom will also help reduce aggression. Don't be afraid to ask for help. Ask others to take your husband for a walk, to the pub, out for lunch, a round of golf... anything to keep him busy and make him tired. You may have friends or find people through your local Alzheimer's organisation or your place of worship who will sit in with your mother or go round there for a cup of tea. Those people are special because they need to understand some unusual or eccentric behaviours, but you can find people who will help you.

8. Use a memory book. There is more about this in the chapter on agitation.

9. To avoid unnecessary stress, do all the things suggested in the first section to keep a calm environment and this may help you to avoid future outbursts. Because it is hard to cope with change when you have dementia, having a routine can be really helpful. Trying to cope with unfamiliar

things can act as a trigger for an aggressive outburst. If you are having outside help, emphasise to them how important it is to have the same faces and the same times, if at all possible. If you are fortunate enough to be able to pay for the help yourself, you can insist on this. Health and social services know that this is important, but sometimes individual managers or workers forget. So remind them.

10. Work out what are the triggers for the person you live with. One of the reasons why families are so successful at caring for each other when one person has dementia is because they know each other really well. You already know what has always been annoying or irritating for each other. You know what pleases each other. When someone goes among strangers, that knowledge would be really useful. So use it when you are caring at home. It is really worth keeping a diary about what is happening. Each day you could say how the person has been. Also make a note of what else happened that day. Over time you may gradually realise that there is a pattern. It might be between not eating enough and getting irritable. If this is the thing, you can plan a snack between meals, and see if it helps. You might realise it always happens after a particular carer has been in. Make sure that you tell them and their manager. Knowledge of the triggers and avoiding them is plain common sense. If you can't see any pattern at all, talk to the doctor about whether there could be something medically wrong or something about the medicines they are taking that could explain it.

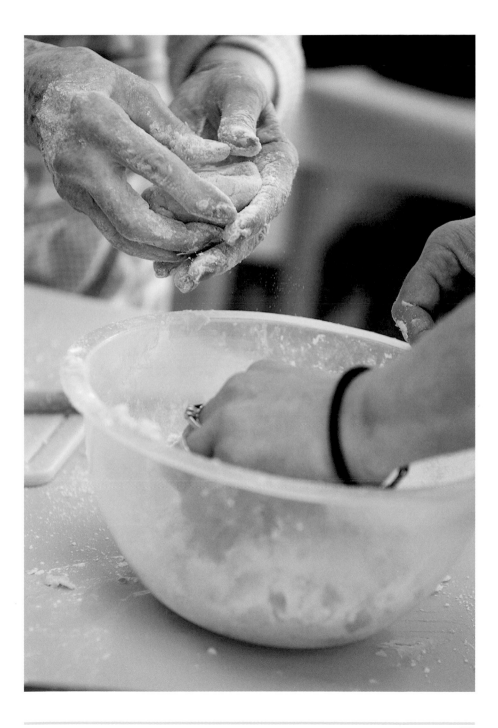

Agitation or Anxiety

When someone is agitated and anxious they are showing their distress, and this is even more distressing for you if you are living with them. If someone you care for is beyond consolation, it clouds your whole existence. In many ways, the strategies for this problem are very like the strategies for aggression. Depending on someone's previous personality, you can predict how they might respond to things they don't like. Some people would react to bad things by being distressed and anxious, and others would react by being angry. That personality might stay the same when they have dementia. You would know whether your husband or wife was the sort of person to react angrily or to bottle things up. The strategies are surprisingly similar.

10 helpful hints for dealing with agitation or anxiety:

1. Protect yourself. It is not like protecting yourself from being bashed by someone, but the emotional bashing from being with an agitated and anxious person all the time is exhausting. They might not be sleeping, so that means you are not sleeping either. You are going to be exhausted. You need to get rest, and remove yourself from some of it. You need to know that it is not your fault, but an expression of the underlying illness. However, you need to remember that you might be able to help yourself by trying to avoid some of the triggers.

2. Ask yourself if there is something physical underlying the distress, and take them to the GP to get it checked out. It is possible to have clinical depression as well as dementia and there are treatments available. Make sure the GP knows what effect it is having on you. You are a patient of that health care team, as well as being the carer for your loved one. It is in their interest to take good care of you, because if you get ill or have to give up they'd have an even bigger job on their hands to care for the person with dementia.

3. Touching and holding the person can be very comforting, but as described in relation to aggression, if the person is pacing about and agitated, trying to restrain them is only likely to make them even more agitated. You know that they will probably fight you, and someone is going to get hurt.

4. Purposeful exercises like a walk or a swim can help burn up the energy that is being channelled into anxiety. It will help the person to sleep better at night. It will improve appetite and also help prevent some of the uncomfortable gastric feelings like sore tummies or constipation.

5. Many people find that aromatherapy or massage is helpful when the person is agitated or anxious. It is astonishing how much this has caught on, even in places like the NHS, where many nurses and care assistants have learned how to do aromatherapy hand massage with essential oils. Of course you have to be careful about the oils, but the dangers will be highlighted by the people who sell them to you. No one really knows if the success of this is to do with the ingredients of the oils or the exact technique of the massage, or the importance of your hands. The most cynical of us knows how nice it can be if someone just sits with you and talks while doing some small kindness. Men find this relaxation at the barber. Ladies usually love going to the hairdresser or for a manicure. This guide is, above everything, pragmatic. So try aromatherapy massage, and if it works, keep on doing it.

6. Again a relaxing environment can help a lot. It is most restful for a person at home if as little as possible is changed. You may make some small changes to make the place safer underfoot, in order to prevent falls. People with dementia who have a fall often end up in hospital and the outcome is not always very good. Getting rid of trip hazards such as mats and old slippers is good. Otherwise the best thing you can do is increase the light levels. It keeps everything else the same, but it is just as if the person's eyesight improved. They can see what they have got and where they are going. This can help to reduce agitation.

7. However, the person may not remember the house as it was this month or last year, but might start looking for things that used to be there. They can be agitated

because they feel they have lost something. They might ask what happened to their favourite chair, when you know that it was thrown away years ago, at their own instigation. They might accuse you of stealing things, or panic about burglars. It stands to reason if they don't remember giving something away, then someone must have taken it. The person is being very logical and intelligent, but just forgot a whole chunk of time.

'My cousin Brigitte believed in ghosts, so when things were not where she remembered leaving them, she assumed she had a poltergeist in the house.'

Having a supernatural thing in the house would make anyone agitated. Arguing about it is not usually going to help, as the person will either become personally undermined, or be reinforced in the idea that you yourself are dishonest. Distraction is the best move. There are hints about distraction throughout this booklet.

8. People who have agitation sometimes seem to benefit from light therapy, or daylight lamps. This is meant to mimic being out in daylight, so again, walking in the open air is good. Keep the curtains wide open and the windows clean and cut away bushes from the view. There is more about daylight lamps in the section on depression.

9. Music is such a good medicine, it should be available on the national health. However, just like other medicines, it needs to be the right music, and you need to know a lot about the person to be able to get the right music for their mood.

10. Life story work. This means working with the person to find out interesting and important things that happened in their life. What is interesting depends on the person. For example, you might think the most interesting thing is that she was the shop steward in her factory after the war, but she might think that the most interesting thing was her child. You might expect her to be more defined by her family, but she may be more defined by some relationship that she has not mentioned for years. Gathering the story together and recording it can be hugely interesting and the activity itself seems to make the person feel better. It is time well spent for most people. There may be some topics that you wish to avoid, but be guided by the person with dementia. You might wish they did not think about things that make them sad, but sometimes a good cry can be very therapeutic. However, it is usually meant to be a fun activity. Not least it allows the person with dementia to give something back to other people, at a time when they must feel as if they are always muddled and getting things wrong. You don't have to make a book, but if you decide to do that, you can write down some of the stories before they get forgotten, and insert pictures and photos if you have any. Then when the person is agitated or anxious, they can sit down with their scrap book and remember happy times. If they have visitors it can be the focus for a discussion. It brings up information about likes and dislikes.

'I always wondered why Papa would never eat chicken and it turns out that his own grandfather had kept them in the yard. Papa would play with them and then his grampa would wring their necks! He told me this story when we were looking at a picture of their old house.'

If you have access to a computer you can create a life story book electronically by visiting www.caringmemories. net, and the book you make can be sent to you in hard back. You can share the electronic version with relatives all over the world, and they often have some new information to offer. Families love it and often order extra copies of the book to keep for themselves. What started as a distraction to reduce agitation becomes a family heirloom.

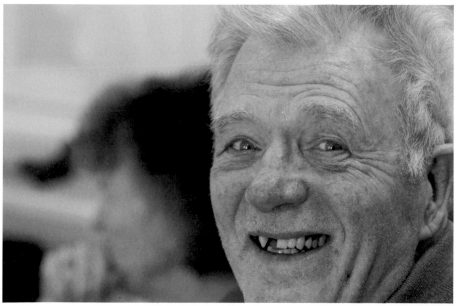

Depression

The person with dementia can suffer from depression on top of their dementia. While they have the depression it can make the dementia symptoms worse so it is always worth treating the depression. Sometimes you have the impression that the dementia got worse, but you can reverse some of that by dealing with the depression. Because health professionals don't always think of depression or spot it, the person you care for is rather dependent on you knowing them and knowing when they are 'down'.

10 helpful things for depression:

1. Activities that relieve boredom or distract the person, which have already been described, may help when they are depressed. Anyone who is bored and inactive is likely to dwell on their problems. You know them well, so you know what would cheer them up.

'When dad gets down, I stick him in the car and we take a run down to the harbour. Just watching the boats coming in and out seems to lift him and he tells stories about when he was in the navy.'

2. Animals are good companions for cheering people up, and they can seem quite sympathetic. No matter how 'down' his master feels, the dog still needs his walk, and maybe the fresh air, exercise, and daylight together will be helpful for those low feelings, both for man and dog.

3. Remembering and reminiscence is very good for depression. You can undertake this in a number of ways. Stick on an old movie, or a favourite documentary that can be talked about. Look over old photographs, or look at the life story book you are working on. You can get other members of the family involved in this. In fact, it is a great way of bringing the generations together.

'We were doing a school project on the Blitz and I even got a part in the show we put on. It turned out that Granny was evacuated from London in the war and went to live in the country with a lady called Vera. She told me so many stories. She did not even have to have any lessons for six months. She says that is why she is no good at spelling now. It is funny though. She keeps calling me Doris and that's my mum's name, but I don't mind.'

Sometimes an old object or item of clothing can help. Imagine the laughter when you are discussing it, again in particular with younger people.

'Your lapels were this wide? And this is meant to be a tie?'
'You used this for making shapes with butter? How hygienic was that? It's wooden.'
'You bashed your clothes with this while washing? No! Really? Good grief!'
'I don't believe it...you had to wear this object to school...? Aagh!'

If you are skilled at this, you can start really good conversation about the past, and take the person out of their gloomy spiral of thoughts.

4. There is research that suggests you can make things better using 'multisensory therapy' which involves stimulating the person with music and light, and even nice smells, to lift them from their depression. You can buy a machine with lights that change and fibre optics strands to play with. In some care homes they have a whole room like this where people lie on cushions and stare at the lights.

5. Validation. One temptation when the person is depressed, is to try to persuade them they are wrong about the fact of what's making them sad.

'Mum was crying as if her mother had died yesterday. Her mum died fifty years ago! I hear dad going on and on at her to remind her that they all went to the funeral before we were even born.'

There is a way of dealing with this called 'validation'. Instead of making her out to be wrong, which is depressing in itself, the thing is to go with the flow of the feelings. You can reply to her crying by saying, 'Oh your mum was lovely wasn't she? Tell me what sort of thing she used to cook for your tea...' The person is not made to feel foolish. It doesn't matter that she was wrong about when her mother died.

The important thing is to give comfort, because it is right to feel grief. Most of us have the comfort that time brings when someone died in the past, but if you have forgotten the passage of that time, the grief is very new, and should be responded to like that.

6. Don't argue if it doesn't matter. You have probably already learned not to correct them if the person with dementia says things which are not true. Correcting people in most of our lives is very useful. It helps children to learn if you correct them. It can help others to get along if you give them advice when they appear to be wrong. However, the person with dementia is going to be wrong very often, and they have difficulty in learning much that is new. So correcting them continuously ends up being exhausting for everyone and depressing for everyone. Drawing attention to the problem can make the person with dementia feel angry and useless, and that can make them depressed as well.

7. Many dementia organisations recommend counselling as a help for depression. The research that has been done so far does not suggest that it makes a major difference, but when you see how often it is recommended, it must be worth trying. At the very least it is a distraction. The counsellor may be offering stimulation and be able to give hints on how to manage the behaviour that the depressed person with dementia exhibits. You need to be sure that they know the person has dementia, as some counselling only works if the person learns new behaviour between sessions, and the person with dementia is not going to be very good at learning.

8. Did we mention exercise? Well, yet again it turns out to be really useful. Depression keeps people awake and exercise helps them to sleep. Exercise gets you out in the daylight and that is really important for chasing away the winter blues. Of course people get depressed in the middle of summer, but it is a well known fact that people get more depressed in the long dark days of winter. Exercise appears to release chemicals in our bodies that make us feel better. But don't do it alone. Exercise in company is the best.

9. Companionship. People with dementia, particularly at the early stages, get a huge amount of support if they are able to take part in a group involving people like themselves. Contact your local Alzheimer's Society to find out if there is one, or ask the community psychiatric nurse if they are going to start one. Dementia support groups are a great place to talk in safety about the things that are of concern. In some cases they even manage to work together to make changes happen in services. Not least they are a place of great happiness.

'I am a professor in the field and I take it all very seriously. The people at the dementia working group, all of whom have dementia, have me rocking with laughter. It is about

dementia, about themselves, about how others treat them. Of course they are angry and sad, but they share their laughter generously and tell me that it is better than any medicine.'

10. As with agitation, remember that you need to look after yourself. If the person you are caring for is beyond consolation, you definitely need to look for help and some of the addresses at the end of this booklet might be useful.

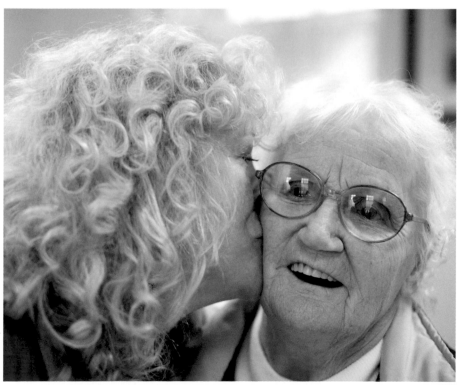

Hallucination

Hallucinations are when people see or hear things that are not there. Sometimes you can look at something and mistake what it is. You might see a shadow and think it is a person. You might 'see' faces in a wallpaper pattern. In these cases it's usually called an 'illusion' – because once the light is improved, or you put your glasses on, you can dismiss it as a misinterpretation of something that is really there. It is there, but it's not what you thought it was.

The person with dementia can sometimes misinterpret an image or picture for the real thing. For example, they might try to pick the leafy pattern off the carpet, thinking that someone has trampled leaves all over the floor.

Another misinterpretation is when someone sees their own face in the mirror, and thinks it is a stranger looking back at them through a window. They don't recognise their own real face, because they would expect their face to be years younger. They may have forgotten their sixties and seventies and think they are still fifty. This is the same problem that makes mothers mistake their son for their husband, and forget that they ever had grandchildren. They might look at their husband and say to their son, *"Who's that old man that keeps hanging round me?"* That mistake is sometimes very hard for families and always very sad. It is important to remember how much you were loved, before the forgetting began. And of course, try not to argue. If you need any reassurance ask, 'What's your husband like?' and watch the love in her face as she describes you. Maybe it's from the past, but it is true.

Hallucinations are different. They are more common in certain types of dementia and they can be made more likely by medication, infections, and other illness. The person may not only see things that are not there – and have never been there – but hear or smell them, or even feel them. Any of the five senses may be confused. The person might hear voices saying bad things. As a result of that the person might become suspicious or frightened.

Depending on how you think about them, or what form they take, hallucinations can be horrible, or just a distraction. Knowing whether your relative is hallucinating can be really helpful in understanding what they are doing and saying. The medical team need to be told about them.

10 helpful hints for coping with hallucinations:

1. Don't argue about whether the voices or sights are there. There is nothing you can say that will make the image go away. It is not a matter of logic so you can't use your reasoning to make it go away. The following exchange is not helpful.
'How could there be a rabbit on the balcony…? Don't be silly! It would fall off. How could it get there?' The person might then start to be distressed with anxiety for the poor rabbit, which you have given more substance to by your comments. It is now a rabbit in danger from his point of view. You don't want the man to rush out to rescue it.

2. Try not to make the person feel more disturbed than they already are, or silly. Telling them off or 'proving' that the hallucination is false will be very hard. It won't work and it will feel bad for both of you.

3. If you suspect it is based on an illusion, try to take the confusion away: put on the light, open the curtains, shed light on the subject. Check it out in case there is something happening. Keep a diary to see if there is a particular pattern of the thing appearing. If there is, you may be able to avoid the triggers. Maybe it happens at a certain time of day. The more information you have to give to the nurse or doctor, the easier it will be to find things that might help.

4. If it is a horrible hallucination, give all the comfort you would give if it was real. If your mum sees a bird and is frightened of birds, shield her and cuddle her and say, 'Don't worry I'll deal with this for you. I'll make it go away.' You are not lying, it is just that you are dealing with it in a way that she may not understand. Your comfort and distraction will 'make it go away'.

5. When dealing with it, use distraction. It has been suggested that the person is more likely to hallucinate if there is no distraction. It appears that some people with dementia will be aware of the hallucination and acknowledge it, but are able to 'tune out' of it – like having the TV on, but not watching it, or having someone in the room to whom you are paying no attention. They are still aware of it, but they screen it out. If there is nothing else to think about, this is harder.

6. Make it less likely to happen by making sure the atmosphere is not boring, but not over stimulating either. It appears that hallucinations are more likely if the person is stressed, for example by coping with changes in routine or carers.

7. Make sure the person has enough to eat and drink, and enough sleep.

8. Ask the pharmacist or the doctor to review the medication regime to make sure that this is not part of the problem. The doctor may also wish to give the person a full examination to make sure there is not any other underlying physical illness that is causing the problem.

9. Don't worry. Some hallucinations can be quite nice, like a bird or flowers. There are worse problems than imagining nice things, as you know. Understanding the cause may make you less worried, and depending on how much insight the person with dementia has, they might be perfectly aware that they are 'seeing things' and consciously coping with it.

10. Remember the squirrel! 'My mum kept saying to me, when I asked her how she was, "Oh don't worry about me, Basil keeps me company. He comes round for afternoon tea." We assumed that she had an imaginary friend because we knew about the hallucinations and she'd had Parkinsons. I wondered if we should tell the doctor. The children even joined in talking about Basil. When I was doing her blinds one day I saw this squirrel on the washing pole and when I pointed it out to her she said, "Of course, that's old Basil. Open the window and he'll come in for his treats."'

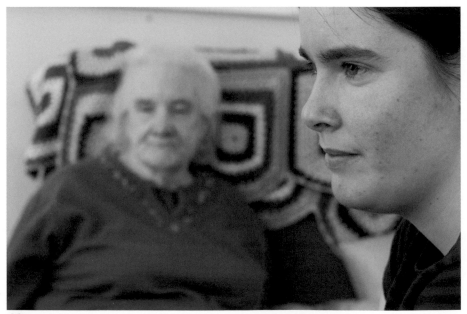

Sleeplessness

It is not for nothing that sleep deprivation is used as a form of torture. Having a decent sleep is important for the person you are caring for. However, you will not last very long if you are not given the chance to have a full night's sleep yourself. People with dementia sleep more lightly, so it is important to make the changes you would need in your house to try to avoid waking them when they have fallen asleep.

10 helpful hints to combat sleeplessness:

1. Exercise is the best way of making someone tired and ensuring a good healthy sleep. Even if it is hard to get out walking, there are things you can do, even from sitting in the chair. Getting out and about, socialising and having a lot of activities to relieve boredom in the day will reduce the likelihood of the person snoozing all day and cruising all night, so being organised and getting help in the day is an important thing to do. You need to make sure the person you want to sleep is tired, so if you can avoid them having too many daytime naps, it's good. Napping is often out of boredom, not tiredness.

2. Have a bedtime routine. It is different for everyone, but may involve a bath, a warm milky drink, winding down by putting off exciting TV or radio programmes, putting on the nightlights, and putting out the cat. Whatever makes the routine most recognisable to the person with dementia as bedtime, should be followed. Does the dog sleep on the bed? Some people find a soft toy comforting at night. Does the person like to fall asleep listening to music? Press the snooze button on the player, so that it switches off after twenty minutes.

3. Put away all daytime things. People get confused about day and night so remove anything that would make them think it IS daytime. Put away the day clothes to reduce the likelihood of the person getting up and dressed in the middle of the night. Some care homes have started issuing staff with dressing gowns for night time, so when the person with dementia wakes up, it is someone who looks like they want to sleep ushering them back to bed and whispering 'Shush! I want to sleep.' Otherwise, with their bright lights and daytime clothes they would make the residents think it is time to get up.

4. Make the bed and bedroom as comfortable as possible. A nice warm bed in a cooler room makes it more likely that the person will stay under the covers.

5. Think about the lighting conditions which are best for your loved one. There may be a need for a small night light to guide the person to the room door or to give reassurance. You can buy a simple device that sticks to the wall with an infrared beam on it. This harmless beam can't be seen in the dark, but when someone passes through it, it can switch on a light. If you put it by the bed, it can be arranged so that it switches on the bathroom light, thus guiding the person to the loo, which is the commonest kind of night time need. If you sleep in a different room, it can be connected to a buzzer under your pillow, which will alert you to the fact that the person you care for is on the move. If you sleep in the same room and bed, you will be all too aware!

6. In an ideal world the head of the bed should be in a position where the person with dementia can see the toilet. This is simpler if you have an en suite bathroom. It also means that if they are in the toilet, they can see the bed and might just go back. If they have to go out into the hall or corridor, the infrared beam that switches on the light in the toilet is very useful. There are more hints about night time wandering in the next section.

7. The person with dementia is likely to be older, and those of us over fifty know that a number of aches and pains may set in after that age. Of course we look after ourselves, haunting the counter at the pharmacy looking for things to rub on our aching limbs, mixtures for our sore throats, tablets for headaches and muscle pains. The person with dementia may have a painful condition about which we are unaware, and it might be a good idea to check this out and make sure that they have had their pain

medication before they go to sleep, so that they have a better chance of a good night. They may have other disorders which cause pain and discomfort such as constipation or a urinary tract infection which causes difficulties. You can get these checked out.

8. While you are at the doctors, check with her and it might turn out that a small alcoholic drink is permitted along with the medication in the evening. A glass of sherry or a half of stout might be just the thing at bedtime. Have a small one yourself! A glass of red wine a day is supposed to help protect you from getting dementia. Have something nice for yourself at the end of the day. Research has shown that the wellbeing of the person taking care of the person with dementia is crucial. You have to look after yourself. People who have a husband or wife with dementia, and who have sleep disturbance as a result, are at risk of getting depression over time. You might think of having a family member to 'sleep over' at your place now and again so you could get proper rest.

9. Snacks may help during the night. I know a man who wakes up craving a banana sandwich at 2am and goes back to sleep contented. If you have got something ready, wrapped in film nearby, you can produce it with the minimum of fuss, before the whole household is awake. No need for bright lights, or rushing about. A slurp of milk and off to sleep again. It makes sense to avoid anything that you know has a lot of caffeine in it, because it does keep people awake. The dentist might not think it is very clever not to brush his teeth, but if it is a choice between that and a sleep, I know which I would vote for.

10. Preventing the person from walking about at night is a problem in itself. For the purpose of this section, the important thing is to get the person you care for to sleep, and help them stay asleep, and get them back to sleep as soon as possible if they wake up. The hints above might help with that, but as you have seen there is nothing magic that can be recommended. The doctor can always offer a sedative if you are at the end of your tether, but this can cause as many problems as it solves. The person might not be fully awake the next day and prone to dozing in the chair, and even falling over. Then the next night as the sun goes down, it all starts over again.

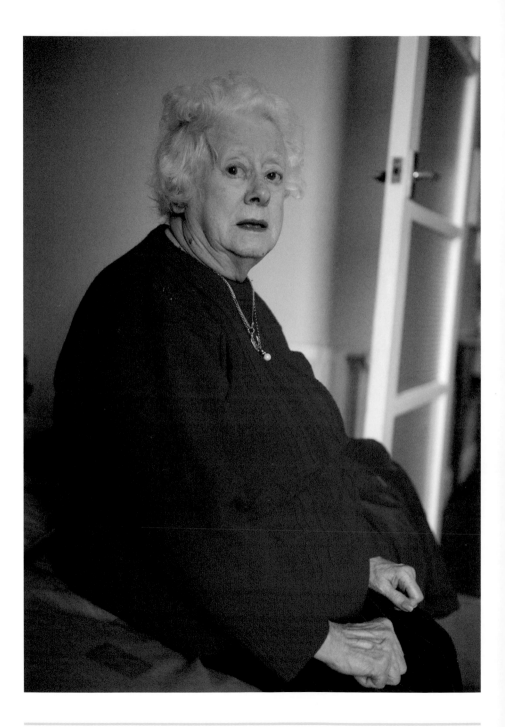

Wandering

The experts spend a lot of time arguing about what to call this behaviour, but it seems that most relatives just call it wandering. What we mean is when the person walks about at a time or in a place where you don't think it is a good idea, perhaps because they are likely to come to harm, or because it seems pointless.

It is a nightmare if the person you care for goes missing. Neighbours and police need to be alerted. The stories go through your mind that you have read in the newspaper about people being found dead. You resolve that if you get them back it will NEVER happen again. The mixture of relief and anger when they return is channelled into trying to make your house into a fortress from which they will not escape. You ask the police about tagging devices. You lock the place up.

Others say that wandering about in the house is very taxing, whether the person is shadowing you from room to room so that you can't even go to the bathroom alone, or pacing back and forward over the same ground.

The practical solutions are based on the different reasons for the walking about behaviour. It might be because the person

- is in pain, and can't tell anyone, and can't sit because of it
- needs the toilet and is confused about what to do
- feels trapped, stressed and anxious and is looking for an exit
- is confused and thinks there is something important (from

the past, like going to work, or collecting the children)
that they must do
- doesn't know where they are and wants to go 'home'
- is bored and frustrated
- finds the repeated movements comforting
- any combination of the above and things we have not
thought of

The solutions include alternatives to wandering, and things
to do to avoid the hazards of wandering.

10 helpful hints for coping with wandering:

1. Check out the underlying reasons, including the
possibility that the person has a physical problem which
could be treated. At the same time, make sure that none
of the medication provided for other conditions could be
causing a problem.

2. Use any of the strategies in the previous sections to
see if the person is bored and frustrated, or is being made
anxious by the atmosphere in the house. This will include
aromatherapy massage, using music, and the multisensory
stimulation of lights for distraction.

3. At the risk of repetition, exercise comes up again as
an important strategy. If the person is tired, they will often

sit down and rest. If they want to walk, take them for a walk or get someone else to do so. There is usually no such thing as bad weather, only the wrong shoes or clothes. In some towns there are 'Walky Talky' clubs where people of a certain age go walking in groups, on relatively easy walks and often round the town. We have heard of one in urban Belfast that is for men only, and they go to the pub at the end until their families come to collect them.

4. When the person is trying to leave, it is not a good idea to try to restrain them. If the reason for leaving is a confused one, they will be determined to do what they set out to do, eg collecting the children from school. It is better to get them to put on the right clothes, and to offer to go with them. You should not try to argue with the person. That only fixes the idea that they need to go. Once going along, you may be able to distract them and they'll relax and return home with you happily.

5. If walking out is impossible other forms of distraction may reduce the tension. Some time spent on the life story work, or looking through the book may help. Music and dancing on the spot may help to burn up some energy.

6. Unwanted exiting from the house can be a nightmare. Of course, you can lock your doors. Distracting the person from trying to get through them can become a problem,

as the locked door becomes a focus of all their attention. It is very important if you decide to use locks, that there is not a fire hazard. You may need to get out in a hurry, so don't make your security so complicated that you can't exit yourself swiftly in an emergency. Sometimes painting a door the same colour as the surrounding wall makes it 'invisible' to a person with dementia so they are less likely to recognise it as being an exit. A large sign saying 'Don't go through this door', though simple, might work, and you can buy signs like this that will light up at night, activated by a movement sensor. Switch off your outside lights at night, to avoid the person going outside towards the light.

7. In case your loved one gets lost, in spite of your best efforts, make sure that they have their identity on them. A card or note in a pocket or bag is good, but sewing something into their clothing can help. If they carry a mobile phone and it is switched on it may be possible to trace them. Families consider tracking devices, so that their loved one can have the freedom to roam, but with the backup of being able to be retrieved if they go too far, or stay away for too long. Identification bracelets can be a good idea.

8. If the person who wanders has some usual haunts, make sure the people know who they are and where they belong. Open an account for your dad at the pub, and tell the staff who to ring if he turns up. Make sure the lady

in the post office knows that if he turns up looking for the family allowance, he's not a rather incompetent fraudster. She will understand. In some communities your neighbours and local businesses are like a neighbourhood watch, and can help.

9. If the person gets lost a recent photograph is very helpful for the search and it is good if you can remember, or work out, what the person was wearing that day. The more people know the better, so details like where they used to work or live, and what habits they have are really useful for working out where to start looking.

10. When they are found again, it is important to relax. No harm has been done, and you are not to blame for them going away. You need to talk to everyone who can help you, including the social work department and your doctor, your family and your local Alzheimer's organisation.

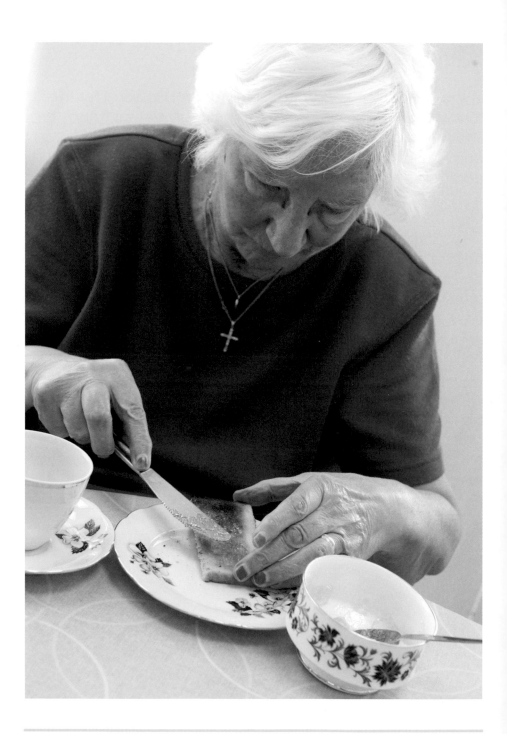

Organisations that can help

This booklet has been written as guidance for people with dementia and their carers. It is based on a larger work, which was a search of the published scientific studies about what actually works. This is available at http://www.leeds.ac.uk/lihs/psychiatry/reports.html

Always remember that help is at hand, through your GP or local social services. In addition here are some other organisations that might help.

Carers UK
20 Great Dover Street
London
SE1 4LX
T: 020 7378 4999
www.carersuk.org

The Princess Royal Trust for Carers
Unit 14, Bourne Court
Southend Road,
Woodford Green
Essex
IG8 8HD
0844 800 4361
www.carers.org

Counsel and Care
Twyman House
16 Bonny Street
London,
NW1 9PG
020 7241 8555
www.counselandcare.org.uk

Alzheimer Scotland
22 Drumsheugh Gardens
Edinburgh
EH3 7RN
0131 243 1453
www.alzscot.org

Alzheimer's Society
Devon House
58 St Katharine's Way
London
E1W 1LB
020 7423 3500
www.alzheimers.org.uk

Age UK
York House
207-211 Pentonville Road
London
N1 9UZ
0800 169 6565
www.ageuk.org.uk

The Relatives and Residents Association
1 The Ivories
6-18 Northampton Street
London
N1 2HY
020 7359 8136
www.relres.org

Carers Scotland
The Cottage
21 Pearce Street
Glasgow
G51 3UT
0141 445 3070
www.carersscotland.org